How To Stop Ringing In Ears And Tinnitus For Good

326 Effective Tips To Cure And Get Relief Of Tinnitus

ADAM COLTON

Published by BizMove
www.bizmove.com

Table of Contents

1. Tinnitus Fact Sheet

Tinnitus is commonly described as a ringing in the ears, but it also can sound like roaring, clicking, hissing, or buzzing. It may be soft or loud, high pitched or low pitched. You might hear it in either one or both ears. Roughly 10 percent of the adult population of the United States has experienced tinnitus lasting at least five minutes in the past year. This amounts to nearly 25 million Americans.

What causes tinnitus?

Tinnitus (pronounced tin-NY-tus or TIN-u-tus) is not a disease. It is a symptom that something is wrong in the auditory system, which includes the ear, the auditory nerve that connects the inner ear to the brain, and the parts of the brain that process sound. Something as simple as a piece of earwax blocking the ear canal can cause tinnitus. But it can also be the result of a number of health conditions, such as:

- Noise-induced hearing loss
- Ear and sinus infections
- Diseases of the heart or blood vessels
- Ménière's disease

- Brain tumors
- Hormonal changes in women
- Thyroid abnormalities

Tinnitus is sometimes the first sign of hearing loss in older people. It also can be a side effect of medications. More than 200 drugs are known to cause tinnitus when you start or stop taking them.

People who work in noisy environments—such as factory or construction workers, road crews, or even musicians—can develop tinnitus over time when ongoing exposure to noise damages tiny sensory hair cells in the inner ear that help transmit sound to the brain. This is called noise-induced hearing loss.

Service members exposed to bomb blasts can develop tinnitus if the shock wave of the explosion squeezes the skull and damages brain tissue in areas that help process sound. In fact, tinnitus is one of the most common service-related disabilities among veterans returning from Iraq and Afghanistan.

Pulsatile tinnitus is a rare type of tinnitus that sounds like a rhythmic pulsing in the ear, usually in time with your heartbeat. A doctor may be able to hear it by pressing a stethoscope against your neck or by placing a tiny microphone inside the ear canal. This kind of tinnitus is most often caused by problems with blood flow in the head or neck. Pulsatile tinnitus also may be caused by brain tumors or abnormalities in brain structure.

Even with all of these associated conditions and causes, some people develop tinnitus for no obvious reason. Most of the time, tinnitus isn't a sign of a serious health problem, although if it's loud or doesn't go away, it can cause fatigue, depression, anxiety, and problems with memory and concentration. For some, tinnitus can be a source of real mental and emotional anguish.

Why do I have this noise in my ears?

Although we hear tinnitus in our ears, its source is really in the networks of brain cells (what scientists call neural circuits) that make sense of the sounds our ears hear. A way to think about tinnitus is that it often begins in the ear, but it continues in the brain.

Scientists still haven't agreed upon what happens in the brain to create the illusion of sound when there is none. Some think that tinnitus is similar to chronic pain syndrome, in which the pain persists even after a wound or broken bone has healed.

Tinnitus could be the result of the brain's neural circuits trying to adapt to the loss of sensory hair cells by turning up the sensitivity to sound. This would explain why some people with tinnitus are oversensitive to loud noise.

Tinnitus also could be the result of neural circuits thrown out of balance when damage in the inner ear changes signaling activity in the auditory cortex, the part of the brain that processes sound. Or it could be the result of abnormal interactions between neural circuits. The neural circuits involved in hearing aren't solely dedicated to processing sound. They also communicate with other parts of the brain, such as the limbic region, which regulates mood and emotion.

What should I do if I have tinnitus?

The first thing is to see your primary care doctor, who will check if anything, such as ear wax, is blocking the ear canal. Your doctor will ask you about your current health, medical conditions, and medications to find out if an underlying condition is causing your tinnitus.

If your doctor cannot find any medical condition responsible for your tinnitus, you may be referred to an otolaryngologist (commonly called an ear, nose, and throat doctor, or an ENT). The ENT will physically examine your head, neck, and ears and test your hearing to determine whether you have any hearing loss along with the tinnitus. You might also be referred to an audiologist who can also measure your hearing and evaluate your tinnitus.

What if the sounds in my ear do not go away?

Some people find their tinnitus doesn't go away or it gets worse. In some cases it may become so severe that you find it difficult to hear, concentrate, or even sleep. Your doctor will work with you to help find ways to reduce the severity of the noise and its impact on your life.

Are there treatments that can help me?

Tinnitus does not have a cure yet, but treatments that help many people cope better with the condition are available. Most doctors will offer a combination of the treatments below, depending on the severity of your tinnitus and the areas of your life it affects the most.

- **Hearing aids** often are helpful for people who have hearing loss along with tinnitus. Using a hearing aid adjusted to carefully control outside sound levels may make it easier for you to hear. The better you hear, the less you may notice your tinnitus. Read the NIDCD fact sheet Hearing Aids for more information.
- **Counseling** helps you learn how to live with your tinnitus. Most counseling programs have an educational component to help you understand

what goes on in the brain to cause tinnitus. Some counseling programs also will help you change the way you think about and react to your tinnitus. You might learn some things to do on your own to make the noise less noticeable, to help you relax during the day, or to fall asleep at night.

- **Wearable sound generators** are small electronic devices that fit in the ear and use a soft, pleasant sound to help mask the tinnitus. Some people want the masking sound to totally cover up their tinnitus, but most prefer a masking level that is just a bit louder than their tinnitus. The masking sound can be a soft "shhhhhhhhhhh," random tones, or music.
- **Tabletop sound generators** are used as an aid for relaxation or sleep. Placed near your bed, you can program a generator to play pleasant sounds such as waves, waterfalls, rain, or the sounds of a summer night. If your tinnitus is mild, this might be all you need to help you fall asleep.
- **Acoustic neural stimulation** is a relatively new technique for people whose tinnitus is very loud or won't go away. It uses a palm-sized device and headphones to deliver a broadband acoustic signal embedded in music. The treatment helps stimulate change in the neural circuits in the brain, which eventually desensitizes you to the tinnitus. The device has been shown to be

effective in reducing or eliminating tinnitus in a significant number of study volunteers.

- **Cochlear implants** are sometimes used in people who have tinnitus along with severe hearing loss. A cochlear implant bypasses the damaged portion of the inner ear and sends electrical signals that directly stimulate the auditory nerve. The device brings in outside sounds that help mask tinnitus and stimulate change in the neural circuits. Read the NIDCD fact sheet Cochlear Implants for more information.
- **Antidepressants and antianxiety drugs** might be prescribed by your doctor to improve your mood and help you sleep.
- **Other medications** may be available at drugstores and on the Internet as an alternative remedy for tinnitus, but none of these preparations has been proved effective in clinical trials.

Can I do anything to prevent tinnitus or keep it from getting worse?

Noise-induced hearing loss, the result of damage to the sensory hair cells of the inner ear, is one of the most common causes of tinnitus. Anything you can do to limit your exposure to loud noise—by moving away from the sound, turning down the volume, or wearing earplugs or earmuffs—will help prevent tinnitus or keep it from getting worse.

What are researchers doing to better understand tinnitus?

Along the path a hearing signal travels to get from the inner ear to the brain, there are many places where things can go wrong to cause tinnitus. If scientists can understand what goes on in the brain to start tinnitus and cause it to persist, they can look for those places in the system where a therapeutic intervention could stop tinnitus in its tracks.

In 2009, the National Institute on Deafness and Other Communication Disorders (NIDCD) sponsored a workshop that brought together tinnitus researchers to talk about the condition and develop fresh ideas for potential cures. During the course of the workshop, participants discussed a number of promising research directions, including:

- **Electrical or magnetic stimulation of brain areas involved in hearing.** Implantable devices already exist to reduce the trembling of Parkinson's disease and the anxieties of obsessive-compulsive disorder. Similar devices could be developed to normalize the neural circuits involved in tinnitus.

- **Repetitive transcranial magnetic stimulation (rTMS).** This technique, which uses a small device placed on the scalp to generate short magnetic pulses, is already being used to normalize electrical activity in the brains of people with epilepsy. Preliminary trials of rTMS in humans, funded by the NIDCD, are helping researchers pinpoint the best places in the brain to stimulate in order to suppress tinnitus. Researchers are also looking for ways to identify which people are most likely to respond well to stimulation devices.

- **Hyperactivity and deep brain stimulation.** Researchers have observed hyperactivity in neural networks after exposing the ear to intense noise. Understanding specifically where in the brain this hyperactivity begins and how it spreads to other areas could lead to treatments that use deep brain stimulation to calm the neural networks and reduce tinnitus.

- **Resetting the tonotopic map.** Researchers are exploring how to take advantage of the tonotopic map, which organizes neurons in the auditory cortex according to the frequency of the sound to which they respond. Previous research has shown a change in the organization of the tonotopic map after exposing the ear to intense noise. By understanding how these changes happen, researchers could develop techniques to bring the map back to normal and relieve tinnitus.

326 Effective Tips To Cure And Get Relief Of Tinnitus

Tinnitus is usually a temporary condition but for some people it becomes a way of life. They find that the incessant noise takes over their life and causes them to constantly suffer. But there is help available if you are willing to try. Take action against tinnitus by trying the tips below.

1. You should try to quit smoking, and avoid being around people who smoke. Cigarette smoke contains benzenes, which have been shown to have a significant effect on blood pressure. High blood pressure, in turn, is often connected to tinnitus. If you can't quit, at least try to cut back and see if that helps.

2. In order to better deal with your tinnitus, try to stay away from loud noise; it will only exacerbate your condition. You may also want to carry earplugs with you in the event that you cannot avoid a noisy situation. If worse comes to worse, you can always use your fingers to block the noise as well.

3. To prevent your tinnitus from keeping you up all night, purchase a white noise generator or a set of white noise CDs. Try out different sounds until you find one that's a good fit for you. Doing this will allow you to concentrate on the white noise rather than your tinnitus, and will help you get a good night's sleep.

4. Try to stay away from stressful situations. Tinnitus often gets worse when you feel anxious, possibly because of how stress affects your blood flow. Do your best to think about what situations may be stressful in advance, and choose to do something else instead, so that you will stay calm.

5. To avoid aggravating your tinnitus further, choose the foods you eat carefully. Salt, caffeine, artificial sweeteners, and sugar, can all make the symptoms of your tinnitus worse. If you don't want to give up all these things, try eliminating them one at a time to find out which one, if any, is causing problems.

6. The saying goes that a good dog is a tired dog, and this holds true for a person that has tinnitus. If you are completely drained by the time you get into bed, you will have a much easier time falling asleep. Exercise can be an effective remedy to lessen the symptoms, and help make your day easier.

7. There is a small chance that reflexology could help a tinnitus sufferer with his or her symptoms. Check for a professional in your area who has reflexology certification, and always ask for references. Check out any references and find out about their work experience, and most importantly, make sure you feel comfortable being treated by them.

8. A helpful method for dealing with tinnitus is to lower the stress levels in your life. When people become tense or anxious, they have a tendency to focus more on their tinnitus. Some techniques which are beneficial in stress reductions are biofeedback, meditation, and exercise. Getting enough sleep each night can also aid in stress reduction.

9. Certain dental problems can cause or worsen tinnitus. Have a dentist look at your teeth and see if there's anything wrong with them. One possible cause may be a problem with your bite alignment. A dentist can check your bite and jaws to determine whether or not this is the cause of your condition.

10. The state of your mouth could actually affect the severity of your tinnitus. Make sure you get all dental issues taken care of and ensure you don't have temporomandibular joint disorder as either of

those can make your symptoms far worse or even create the problem altogether when you don't have tinnitus at all!

11.   Determining what has caused your tinnitus can be quite a challenge, since there are a number of factors that can lead to the development of this condition. After speaking to several doctors, try to find treatments that can reduce your condition's severity, while learning all you can about the condition. With your symptoms under control, you can work more effectively towards identifying the root cause of the condition.

12.   Exercise is a great way to fight tinnitus because it will exhaust your body. Sp when it comes time to go to sleep, your body will need the rest. Tinnitus symptoms can seem elevated at night when things are quiet and if your body is not tired, this can lead to tossing and turning for hours before you fall asleep.

13.   For relief of your tinnitus, you should try to reduce the amount of caffeine and salt that you consume, or eliminate it altogether. Salt will increase and elevate blood pressure levels and caffeine will stimulate an increase in heart rate. Both of which can increase the tinnitus levels and cause you discomfort.

14. Put a high priority on healthy lifestyle choices-- sleep right, eat right, and stay fit. Sleep for at least eight hours a night, eat a variety of healthy foods and exercise at least five days a week. Tinnitus sufferers can manage their condition much more effectively if they take proper care of themselves. Maintaining the basics of a healthy lifestyle goes a long way to staving off tinnitus symptoms.

15. Live your life with an abundance of hope. For someone battling with tinnitus, a chronic condition that leaves your head in a constant state of "noise," your outlook can be very distressing. Hope gives you something to believe in long term, which allows you to feel better both mentally and physically.

16. If you have trouble falling asleep due to tinnitus then you need to alter your environment to be more sleep-inducing. Install light-blocking drapes, cover up any lights on electronics, and use an item that gives off white noise like a standing fan or a machine which plays sounds like thunderstorms.

17. To help you treat Tinnitus, maintain a low stress level and relax more! It has been shown that stress and anxiety can aggravate or even cause the symptoms of Tinnitus. By learning to relax and

controlling your stress, you can alleviate the symptoms and improve the condition.

18.   There are many herbal remedies which can make tinnitus symptoms reduce to the point that you will forget you have it. Examples are bayberry bark, goldenseal, hawthorn leaf, and myrrh gum. Burdock root is my personal favorite and has given me many years of total relief, sparing me from going crazy in a silent room!

19.   Reduce your intake of caffeine and salt. Caffeine is a stimulant that not only increases your heart rate but also elevates tinnitus levels. Salt acts similarly by elevating blood pressure and increasing aggravating noise levels in your head. Making dietary changes will reduce tinnitus levels and help you get a better night's sleep.

20.   Consider that the source of the ringing in your ears might actually be a problem in your mouth. Have your teeth thoroughly looked at and fix any dental issues. Make sure that any braces, retainers or dentures fit perfectly well and are not tensing muscles further up the head or causing never pains or pinches.

21.   If you have been formally diagnosed with tinnitus, you may be able to decrease its effects by

practicing common relaxation techniques. An individual who is placed under a great deal of stress often finds that his or her tinnitus becomes far more intense as a result. Try controlled breathing, stretching, or meditation to avoid making the ringing worse.

22.   Make sure you don't have any dental problems. See a dentist and make sure you don't have temporo-mandibular joint disease, or any kind of dental or jaw problem that could be causing your tinnitus. In some cases, taking care of dental issues could alleviate any tinnitus you might be experiencing.

23.   Getting enough rest is very important if you suffer from tinnitus. Do not let yourself get rundown and overtired. Without a full night's rest of eight hours, you will find tinnitus attacks more frequent and harder to overcome.

24.   If you suffer from pulsatile tinnitus (the sound in your ears keeps rhythm with your heart) ask your doctor if using tricyclic antidepressants may be beneficial for your condition. These medications have been proven to offer relief to numerous people who suffer from pulsatile tinnitus. Since this class of medication may cause side effects, your

physician may prescribe these drugs only on a trial basis to see if they are effective.

25.   If your tinnitus is getting you down you should instead focus on what's great about your life. Write a list of everything you love, enjoy doing, or are happy you are involved in. This will perk up your spirits and help you to get over the misery tinnitus can bring.

26.   The state of your mouth could actually affect the severity of your tinnitus. Make sure you get all dental issues taken care of and ensure you don't have temporomandibular joint disorder as either of those can make your symptoms far worse or even create the problem altogether when you don't have tinnitus at all!

27.   Avoiding stress is a great way to keep your tinnitus symptoms at a minimum, but an even better technique is to learn how to cope with stress when it comes up. I like to step back and look at the situation as if I was a third party, analyzing it and deciding whether or not it's worth my tinnitus acting up. It usually isn't!

28.   Many people have found relief from their chronic tinnitus from taking nutritional supplements and herbal alternatives. Although

there is almost no scientific evidence to back up these claims, people have found some relief using vitamin B complex, mineral supplements with calcium, magnesium, zinc, and herbal extracts like ginkgo biloba.

29.   The link between tinnitus and physiological distress requires that a multidimensional approach be used when treating the symptoms of tinnitus. Patient education and coping skills could be necessary to alleviate the anxiety that tinnitus can cause. Anxiety and stress are common causes of tinnitus and the worry and stress of it can cause it to worsen over time.

30.   Pulsatile tinnitus is noises in the ears that causes noise that pulsates, as in the beating of the heart. This type of tinnitus is common in pregnant women due to increased blood volume and flow during pregnancy. The good news is that it will go away after the baby is born. Meanwhile, try meditation for relaxation and focus away from the noise.

31.   Children are often bothered by tinnitus and ringing in their ears. This is often due to a sinus infection or an ear infection. Ensure your child gets the right treatment. You should then explain what

these noises are and how they will dissipate as the ear infection is treated.

32.   Use caution when evaluating tinnitus remedies. Some vendors offer treatments such as mega-vitamin therapies or herbal medications, but these products may not work for everyone. If you decide to try an alternative remedy, discuss it with a pharmacist first, and only buy a small amount to test before making a larger financial commitment. This can help you avoid wasting money on ineffective or unsafe treatments.

33.   Reducing your stress levels can be all that it takes to get rid of tinnitus. High levels of stress can cause a variety of different medical conditions, with tinnitus being one of them. So, controlling your levels of stress can also reduce or get rid of chronic ringing in your ears.

34.   Research the various natural remedies for tinnitus. There are many means that people were able to successfully treat tinnitus for centuries without the use of medication. Be sure to talk with your physician before trying something, as some herbs can interact with medication, and some of the options available may not be healthy for you.

35.   To get a restful night's sleep even with tinnitus, work out before bedtime. Exercise will tire your body out, and will leave you so exhausted that you'll be able to drift off to sleep peacefully without focusing on your tinnitus. Taking a hot bath after your workout can make falling asleep even easier.

36.   Some who suffer from tinnitus report symptom relief after trying reflexology; try it out to see if it helps you. Locate an accredited professional with references available. Look at their experience and pick out a person that you feel is trustworthy.

37.   To help you cope with tinnitus you should avoid stressful situations. Long periods of stress will make the tinnitus noises much louder than they would be if you are in relaxed state. So to help manage your tinnitus and not make it worse, you should try and live your life with the least amount of stress.

38.   To reduce the inner-ear noises associated with tinnitus, use masking devices commonly knownn as white noise devises or retraining therapy. For some people, masking devices can cover the noise in the ears rendering it less noticeable. Retraining therapy for tinnitus involves the use of psychological counseling to aid those suffering from tinnitus to adapt to their condition.

39. Do you have a ringing, hissing, roaring or buzzing sound in your ears that seems to beat in time with your heart? You could possibly be suffering from a condition known as pulsatile tinnitus. Seek advice from your doctor to determine if you are suffering from this condition. Some things that can cause pulsatile tinnitus are excessive ear wax, exposure to loud noises and the stiffening of the bones in the inner ears. By determining the cause for your tinnitus, your physician may be able to help relieve it.

40. If you are one of the unlucky people that suffer from tinnitus and you have noticed an increase in the severity of it, you may want to have your blood pressure checked. High blood pressure has proven to be one of the causes for increasing severity of tinnitus. If it is high, find ways to lower it.

41. Be aware of your unfinished business throughout the early part of the day and try not to leave anything too important on your plate. That way, when you lay down at night, your tinnitus won't be aggravated while you are consumed in thoughts about what you failed to complete throughout the previous day.

42.   It is vitally important to let your family doctor know if you're taking any supplements, especially if you're on any prescription drugs. The interaction between supplement and prescription can actually bring on the symptoms of tinnitus, so give your doctor a list of any vitamins, herbs, or homeopathics you're taking.

43.   Finding a support group for sufferers of tinnitus is a great way to be surrounded by people who understand what you're going through. If you can't find one locally you can always join a group online or start posting on a tinnitus forum. You'll find both medical professionals and your peers, and they'll all have valuable information you can use.

44.   Do not believe that there is nothing to be done for your tinnitus. If your physician tells you that you will just have to learn to live with it, it is time to find another doctor. New research in the field is offering the medical community a better understanding of tinnitus and new ideas for its treatment.

45.   Sometimes tinnitus will keep people awake at night because their brain will focus on the noise in their head. They can find comfort in practicing deep relaxation techniques to calm the mind. If they sit in a dark room and imagine themselves

lying on a beach with the waves crashing, sometimes they will wake up in the morning and not even remember trying to fall asleep.

46.   Exercise outdoors whenever you can. Exercise helps to reduce emotional stress; lower stress levels, in turn, can help ease tinnitus symptoms. Being outdoors also surrounds you with nature sounds, which are usually relaxing and also help to mask tinnitus noises. Furthermore, the improvement that exercise can bring to your overall health and quality of life helps to counteract the depression that commonly accompanies chronic conditions like tinnitus.

47.   For an instant and anywhere method to relieve tinnitus, learn conscious breathing techniques. Yoga has a tradition called pranayama, and many oriental mind-body disciplines also have breathing techniques you can learn. When you focus your mind on your breath, the attentions of both your mind and ears are focused on something other than tinnitus.

48.   Once you have secured a little relief from the ringing of tinnitus, you must try to find out why you have tinnitus. It your tinnitus is something that just showed up one day, you might be able to really narrow it down. It is virtually impossible to stop

symptoms from occurring, if you do not know what the cause of them are. Explore any and all possibilities in your effort to find a solution.

49.   Seek advice from a doctor if you are suffering from tinnitus. Tinnitus is likely a sign of a different problem that will likely need treatment from a professional. Chronic tinnitus can also be stressful and make it hard to enjoy a normal day. Tinnitus is unlikely to be deadly, but the benefit of seeing a doctor is that it may be treatable.

50.   If you smoke, you should quit. Smoking narrows all of your blood vessels. When the blood vessels that bring blood to your ears and head are narrowed, it can make tinnitus worse. If you quit, you will be able to deal with tinnitus better. Not only that, but your health overall will be better, which helps any other health conditions you have.

51.   To help you treat Tinnitus, maintain a low stress level and relax more! It has been shown that stress and anxiety can aggravate or even cause the symptoms of Tinnitus. By learning to relax and controlling your stress, you can alleviate the symptoms and improve the condition.

52.   If you suffer from tinnitus, you should consider taking ginkgo biloba. Ginkgo biloba naturally

improves your circulation and can relieve the impact of your tinnitus symptoms. Be sure to investigate the right dose for you. If you take medication, make sure that there is no risk of an adverse reaction.

53.   Consider that the source of the ringing in your ears might actually be a problem in your mouth. Have your teeth thoroughly looked at and fix any dental issues. Make sure that any braces, retainers or dentures fit perfectly well and are not tensing muscles further up the head or causing never pains or pinches.

54.   Consult a good physician. At the first sign of tinnitus, you should be concerned enough to get a proper diagnosis. Only a certified physician can tell you for sure what you're dealing with. Tests can also be run to see if there are any health issues that could be responsible for the tinnitus.

55.   Be sure to let your doctor know right away if you have had a diagnosis of tinnitus in the past. There are as many as 200 different over-the-counter and prescription medications that can exacerbate your condition. By gently providing reminders to your physician about your affliction, you can prevent them from mistakenly prescribing a medicine known to have tinnitus as a side effect.

56.   Use a properly fitted medical device to help relieve tinnitus. A hearing aid alleviates symptoms in about half of tinnitus patients who also have hearing loss. A "tinnitus masker," a device worn in the ear which produces a low-level noise that helps cover the unpleasant ringing sensation, can also benefit patients without hearing loss.

57.   One way to eliminate the stress associated with tinnitus is to repeat your favorite poem. You can do this in your own head or you can scream it from the mountaintops. Have a few favorite poems on hand and repeat them over and over until you feel better and more adequately equipped to do what you need to do.

58.   Quite often tinnitus is caused by age-related hearing loss. Since hearing gets worse as a person gets older, things do not work the way they used to in that area. Then these hearing loss issues can lead to the ringing in the ear. Once you are getting close to sixty, it is a good idea to have your hearing checked regularly.

59.   There could possibly be a variety of medical conditions that could be causing your tinnitus. If you have ruled out all the common causes, you should have your doctor take a look at you and see

if you have any other symptoms for other health conditions. Some ailments that could be a cause include: malformation of capillaries, Miniere's disease, and acoustic neuroma. If you happen to have one of these conditions, your doctor may be able to help you with them.

60.   Although there is limited proof that this in fact works, many people who suffer from tinnitus have stated that various forms of alternative medicine has made a difference for them. Things you might want to consider include: acupuncture, hypnosis, the herb ginkgo, zinc supplements, or lipoflavonoid. Be sure to check with your doctor though before taking a variety of supplements.

61.   Go see your dentist. Your tinnitus could be linked to a dental problem. It may also be because of a problem with your skull or jaw. Make sure you discuss tinnitus as your doctor may be able to assist you. If your tinnitus is due to physical problems, seek help and get that taken care of.

62.   Take a walk to put your tinnitus at bay. Distraction can be a very effective tactic when you are trying to live with the constant ringing in the ears. Walking can help in relieving the symptoms you are experiencing. Try a stroll along a shoreline or in the wind to increase the effectiveness.

63.   It is important to remain calm when facing tinnitus. Remember that rarely does tinnitus signify a serious medical problem and may simply be the ordinary sounds of the processes of your body. Consult a physician in the field of audiology or an ear, nose, and throat doctor to discuss your condition.

64.   You might want to consider learning to play a musical instrument as a way to relieve your tinnitus. Your mind can be tricked into ignoring the ringing from tinnitus when other, more pleasant, sounds are dominant. Try learning to play an instrument that you enjoy hearing. You could pick a guitar, violin, or even a flute. Remember to wear earplugs if you will be playing loudly.

65.   Stay away from situations where there are loud noises. If you cannot, then try using earplugs. A lot of the time tinnitus is created by the exposure you have to loud noises. In order to prevent your tinnitus from worsening, you have to protect your ears from further damage. This is also an effective way to stave off attacks, if you already have tinnitus.

66.   If you have that constant ringing in your ear that is caused by tinnitus, it is important to see a

physician to get a proper diagnosis. Tinnitus can be caused by a variety of sources such as head injuries, ear infections, loud noises, stress, vascular problems, and the side effects of medication. The treatment prescribed for tinnitus will be dependent upon what is causing the condition.

67.   Try to stay away from stressful situations. Tinnitus often gets worse when you feel anxious, possibly because of how stress affects your blood flow. Do your best to think about what situations may be stressful in advance, and choose to do something else instead, so that you will stay calm.

68.   Learn Pilates. Pilates can help you handle your stress, which is one of the things that makes tinnitus worse. If you are able to figure out how to deal with situations that make you anxious, you will feel more freedom to do the things that you love without the fear of exacerbating your condition.

69.   There are many herbal remedies which can make tinnitus symptoms reduce to the point that you will forget you have it. Examples are bayberry bark, goldenseal, hawthorn leaf, and myrrh gum. Burdock root is my personal favorite and has given me many years of total relief, sparing me from going crazy in a silent room!

70.   To get a restful night's sleep even with tinnitus, work out before bedtime. Exercise will tire your body out, and will leave you so exhausted that you'll be able to drift off to sleep peacefully without focusing on your tinnitus. Taking a hot bath after your workout can make falling asleep even easier.

71.   If tinnitus causes you problems when you're trying to fall asleep, consider relaxation techniques. Meditation, deep breathing, and even yoga can help you to get your body completely relaxed so you can overcome the noise in your ears. I personally like to use deep breathing, because it helps me both forget the sound and also keeps my blood pressure low.

72.   There is a saying that good dog is one that is tired, and this thought can also be applied to an individual with tinnitus. If you are exhausted and sleepy at bedtime, it will be easier for you to get a good night's sleep. Exercise can also help reduce the symptoms of tinnitus, making your day easier to get through.

73.   Stop and listen to your home to see what white noise you hear, then use it to help you to cover up the sounds in your ears due to tinnitus. For example, in your room, open the window to see if there's sounds outside that will cover over the ringing in your ears.

74.   If you suffer from tinnitus, you can find great relief in relaxation techniques if you participate in them a few times a day. Lowering your blood pressure and relieving stress can help to reduce the volume of the sound in your ears, thereby helping you to rest, especially at bedtime.

75.   To get your mind off tinnitus, create an alternate noise to listen to. Recite poetry or mantras to yourself. Play a musical instrument. You can even chew gum. Singing and humming your favorite songs is always a pleasant way to get through your day and your mind off of the ringing.

76.   Many ingredients that are found in popular foods and medications have been shown to irritate the hearing cells. One such ingredient is caffeine, which is a stimulant found in abundance in coffee, sodas, and even in chocolate. By avoiding excessive intake of these caffeinated products, an individual can reduce his or her risk of developing tinnitus or other hearing-related symptoms.

77.   Be aware of your unfinished business throughout the early part of the day and try not to leave anything too important on your plate. That way, when you lay down at night, your tinnitus won't be aggravated while you are consumed in

thoughts about what you failed to complete throughout the previous day.

78.   Visit a hearing specialist. Your primary doctor should be able to refer you to a doctor who specializes in the ear and hearing. This medical professional will give you more information about what is physically happening and how you might be able to treat the tinnitus. It might be as simple as removing wax buildup, for example.

79.   Research has shown that stress, and depression has an effect on tinnitus. So if you happen to be feeling stressed out, try to take up yoga or anything that would help you alleviate some of the stress you are experiencing. If you have been feeling depressed, try to see what you can do to help yourself out of that funk. Sometimes changing your daily routine around could work, while at other times you might need your doctor's help.

80.   There could possibly be a variety of medical conditions that could be causing your tinnitus. If you have ruled out all the common causes, you should have your doctor take a look at you and see if you have any other symptoms for other health conditions. Some ailments that could be a cause include: malformation of capillaries, Miniere's disease, and acoustic neuroma. If you happen to

have one of these conditions, your doctor may be able to help you with them.

81.   If you suffer from frequent ringing in the ears, be sure to speak with your doctor about the medications that you are taking. Many people do not realize that a variety of different medications can cause tinnitus. If your medication is the cause, you may want to consider switching medications.

82.   Since many people are not knowledgeable about tinnitus and the problems that it causes for people who suffer from this condition, it is important to educate your family, co-workers and friends about your situation. Inform them about the different conditions and settings that cause you the most problems. Also, ask them for their support in helping you deal with your condition.

83.   Research some relaxation techniques, such as deep breathing or meditation. For many people, being stressed can make the tinnitus worse, and the tinnitus itself causes you stress. This positive feedback loop can be broken through the use of relaxation techniques, which can help reduce the incidents of tinnitus in your life.

84.   Some people elect to try alternative forms of therapy to help them cope with tinnitus. Using the

herb ginkgo biloba on a daily basis can aid in relieving some of these symptoms. For some, alternative therapies such as acupuncture, reflexology and relaxation have proved to be beneficial for tinnitus.

85.   Reduce your intake of caffeine and salt. Caffeine is a stimulant that not only increases your heart rate but also elevates tinnitus levels. Salt acts similarly by elevating blood pressure and increasing aggravating noise levels in your head. Making dietary changes will reduce tinnitus levels and help you get a better night's sleep.

86.   If you are newly experiencing tinnitus, your best approach may be to simply ignore it. The majority of the cases of tinnitus go away on their own. Even if they don't, they subside enough that they do not disrupt your life. If the tinnitus continues to be a problem, however, you should consult your doctor.

87.   Think about life's many stresses if you're interested in freedom from tinnitus. While a physical affliction, tinnitus is often just the manifestation of something emotional. Pay close attention to your schedule and see what you might be affecting your mood. Try a few deep relaxation techniques, and then incorporate the most effective ones into your daily life.

88.   Look for a local or online support group with others who have tinnitus. No matter how much your friends and family try to be supportive, there is nothing to compare with someone who really understands what living with tinnitus is like because they have it, too. When you join a support group, you will find you can share tips and ideas with others who are living through the same experiences you are.

89.   Try using headphones if you cannot drown out the noise from your tinnitus with a radio or television. This directs sound into your ears to cancel tinnitus noise. If you turn up the volume too loud, you can cause further damage.

90.   Keep a diet diary with entries on what you eat, what you crave, and what exercise you engage in, and see if your tinnitus has any relation to any of those factors. Often food allergies can make tinnitus worse, or certain activities can aggravate the symptoms later on in the day.

91.   Use nature to help you with tinnitus. There are many tapes, compact disks, and MP3s filled with nature sounds. Go ahead and get some of the ocean, rain forest, or a waterfall sounds. These will help distract your brain from the discomfort of ear

ringing. Choose your favorite nature sounds and give it a try.

92.   Be patient when beginning a new treatment for tinnitus. Many treatments require some time before they start working and for results to become apparent. In the meantime, make an effort to eliminate sources of stress in your life as it can often cause the symptoms of tinnitus to become more severe.

93.   Understand which sounds you are hearing with your tinnitus. Read up on information provided by medical professionals who study the condition. Learning more about your condition should take the stress and the fear away. Stress and fear work together, and getting rid of the fear is a crucial step to recovery.

94.   You may find that supplementing your diet with minerals or other natural supplements may help to reduce your tinnitus symptoms. Some sufferers of tinnitus have found relief by taking magnesium or zinc. Others have found that Gingko Bilbao minimizes their suffering. Try each one individually so that you can ascertain which works best in your particular situation.

95.   An interesting technique to add to your arsenal in the fight against tinnitus is biofeedback therapy. Often used to help patients reduce their reactions to stress, biofeedback therapy teaches the individual to control certain bodily functions, including their pulse. Many people have discovered that their tinnitus symptoms decrease as they learn to reduce their muscular tension and regulate their skin temperature.

96.   Pulsatile tinnitus is noises in the ears that causes noise that pulsates, as in the beating of the heart. This type of tinnitus is common in pregnant women due to increased blood volume and flow during pregnancy. The good news is that it will go away after the baby is born. Meanwhile, try meditation for relaxation and focus away from the noise.

97.   A good way to help your tinnitus symptoms is to eat a healthy, low sodium diet. If your diet is consistently unhealthy, your body will begin to lack the ability to cure itself. If this goes on too long, it can quickly lead to the development of maladies such as tinnitus.

98.   If you suffer from tinnitus, it can be helpful to find a support group to join. By mingling with people in a support group, you will be surrounded

by others who truly understand the issues associated with having this condition. People in this group can offer compassion and different coping strategies which they have discovered to be helpful to them.

99.   It is important to watch what you eat if you have tinnitus. Believe it or not, certain foods, like those that contain a lot of salt, sugar or artificial sweeteners, can worsen your symptoms. For more information on which foods are beneficial for tinnitus patients, speak with a medical professional.

100. Remain calm. Tinnitus is only rarely a symptom of a serious brain condition or hearing problem. You don't need to stress about suddenly having developed a brain tumor or puncturing an eardrum. Generally, tinnitus is a condition all on its own, without an underlying medical explanation that could lead to other problems.

101. If you believe you might be afflicted with Tinnitus, but you're over 50 you should ask your doctor to test you for Meniere's Disease. This syndrome can afflict you with the same symptoms that Tinnitus can but is far more serious, therefore, a diagnosis is important to help treat it before it gets worse!

102. The ringing in your ears caused by tinnitus can keep you up late at night, but technology can help. There are many white noise generators which provide a variety of sounds for you to listen to, from a rainstorm to nighttime in a forest, which can drown out the sound in your ears.

103. To keep tinnitus from driving you crazy, project it out into the room. Visually pick some corner or object in the room you are in and mentally associate that as the source of the sound. If you pretend that it is not within you, then you can mentally relax that there is nothing wrong with you. This improves your mood and blood pressure.

104. See a doctor immediately if you experience any tinnitus warning signs. Tinnitus occurring in only one ear or accompanied by difficulty swallowing or speaking, severe dizziness, or severe headaches can be a sign of a serious medical problem. Getting prompt diagnosis and treatment in such cases might save your hearing from permanent damage.

105. To reduce the inner-ear noises associated with tinnitus, use masking devices commonly knownn as white noise devises or retraining therapy. For some people, masking devices can cover the noise in the ears rendering it less noticeable. Retraining therapy for tinnitus involves the use of psychological

counseling to aid those suffering from tinnitus to adapt to their condition.

106. When you are diagnosed with a condition such as tinnitus, it is important that you research it and understand it. Make sure to take notes about what triggers tinnitus in you and seek ways of making it more bearable. Even if the doctor claims that your condition will never go away, rest assured that there are constant improvements in the medical field and there are new cures out there waiting to be discovered.

107. You may find some relief from tinnitus if you just find a good masking noise to listen to. This noise could be a ticking clock, static from an unturned radio or an unturned TV channel. The quieter your surroundings are, the more the noises of tinnitus are going to bother you.

108. Tinnitus can be affected by the amount of salt that a person consumes on a regular basis. If you suffer from tinnitus and you notice that the severity of it has increased, you should be sure to cut the amount of salt that you are consuming. The salt will impair blood circulation and make things worse for you.

109. Were you recently in an accident of any kind? Tinnitus has been linked to head or neck injuries because these can affect your inner ear, hearing nerves or even your brain function that is linked to hearing. If you think your tinnitus was affected by a recent injury or accident, try to get it treated as soon as possible to help alleviate some of the ringing you keep hearing.

110. Use background noise to forget about tinnitus. You could leave your TV or radio on, or even hum and sing yourself. Covering the ringing noise will quickly become a habit, and you will soon not even think about tinnitus anymore and simply drown it in other noises. You should be careful about the volume of your background noise.

111. When your tinnitus prevents you from concentrating on your work, listen to music. Make sure you choose music with no lyrics and a calm mood so that it fades into the background and doesn't break your concentration. Soothing music will calm the tinnitus, while also allowing you to concentrate on the task at hand.

112. The many possible causes of tinnitus can make determining the source of your tinnitus difficult. Check with a few doctors and then try to figure out tinnitus treatments that will minimize your

symptoms. Educate yourself on this condition and how it can impact your life. Once you have the symptoms under control, you can return your focus to the cause.

113. Look into some natural sleep aids that can help you fall asleep at night with your tinnitus. Many of the natural sleep aids are not addictive and can help you sleep in spite of the sounds of your tinnitus. If the natural aids do not work, talk to your doctor about a safe sleep aid you can use.

114. It is important to watch what you eat if you have tinnitus. Believe it or not, certain foods, like those that contain a lot of salt, sugar or artificial sweeteners, can worsen your symptoms. For more information on which foods are beneficial for tinnitus patients, speak with a medical professional.

115. Remain calm. Tinnitus is only rarely a symptom of a serious brain condition or hearing problem. You don't need to stress about suddenly having developed a brain tumor or puncturing an eardrum. Generally, tinnitus is a condition all on its own, without an underlying medical explanation that could lead to other problems.

116. Food allergies can cause symptoms which mimic tinnitus, so watching what you're eating or drinking

when your symptoms are at their worst is a great idea to help you deal with the condition. For example, caffeine is known to cause ringing in the ears, vertigo, and other tinnitus-like symptoms in some people.

117. The ringing in your ears caused by tinnitus can keep you up late at night, but technology can help. There are many white noise generators which provide a variety of sounds for you to listen to, from a rainstorm to nighttime in a forest, which can drown out the sound in your ears.

118. Avoid alcohol, caffeine and tobacco if you are a sufferer of tinnitus. These substances are known to act as nerve stimulants. Tinnitus is often caused by over-stimulated nerves sending a confused message to the brain, so adding to this is naturally something you should avoid. Removing these will also help your overall health, so their is no reason not to.

119. Consider seeking help from a psychologist if you suffer from tinnitus. A psychologist has the ability to teach you how to put the tinnitus to the back of your mind. To do this you must be fully cooperative with the psychology and open your mind to the fact that this can work for you.

120.   Call your primary care physician. You need to get a proper diagnosis so it will ease your worries. Only a certified physician can tell you for sure what you're dealing with. He can run tests to rule out other health problems that could cause or contribute to your tinnitus.

121.   Multiple studies have shown that elevated levels of blood fats may cause serious and permanent inner-ear malfunction that is accompanied by ringing in the ears. Follow a diet plan that is low in fat; avoid fatty meats, cheeses, fried snacks, and over-processed baked goods. It is not enough to simply avoid trans fats; to protect the health of your ears, you should limit consumption of all kinds of fats.

122.   Be patient with your treatments for tinnitus. There any many different routes out there that you can take, but you want to give each one sufficient time to do its' job. Don't give up on a treatment until you've tried it for a significant amount of time. Some treatments take longer than other for their outcomes to really be noticed.

123.   Think about seeing a therapist. If tinnitus is causing stress in your life, seeking out a therapist to talk about ways to decrease stress is probably a good idea. By decreasing stress in other areas of

your life, tinnitus will be easier to cope with; a therapist can help you with that.

124. Have your doctor or audiologist recommended a support group or forum for you. By sharing some of the issues you are having with tinnitus with others who have the same thing, it could help you alleviate some of the stress you feel from it. You may also learn some coping techniques that others have used to help them get through it.

125. With a good massage, your body can relax, your mind can clear, your blood flows freely, and you should notice less tinnitus. When you're relaxed, your heart won't have to work so hard, which will cause your blood pressure to go down. In a few tinnitus cases, the tinnitus sound is simply blood rushing through the ears, so in these cases, slowing down the blood flow can relieve the symptoms.

126. After you have been diagnosed with tinnitus, you must enlist the support of a qualified team of medical professionals. Your doctor may refer you to an audiologist, or perhaps to another specialist.

127. Take a walk to put your tinnitus at bay. Distraction can be a very effective tactic when you are trying to live with the constant ringing in the ears. Walking can help in relieving the symptoms

you are experiencing. Try a stroll along a shoreline or in the wind to increase the effectiveness.

128. Avoiding situations which aggravate the symptoms of your tinnitus is an effective strategy to keeping it under control. Stay away from loud noises, stress, caffeine, and sodium-rich foods to avoid triggering your symptoms. Engage in exercise daily to help keep your blood pressure in check and your body healthy to reduce symptoms.

129. Develop a habitual pattern of exercise, diet and sleep. Exercise several times per week, consume a healthy diet and get proper rest every day. All of these are excellent stress-management techniques for tinnitus sufferers, as the condition can be stressful. Despite the tinnitus, being able to manage the basics can improve life.

130. It's extremely important for you to alter the way you treat your ears so that your tinnitus doesn't get any worse! Avoid listening to music at high volume through earbuds, and wear earplugs when engaging in any loud work. You'll want to buy high quality earplugs, not foam, for maximum protection.

131. Talk to your doctor about getting a blood test to check your zinc level. In people with low levels, zinc supplements have been shown to help many

with their tinnitus. High levels of zinc supplements must be monitored by a doctor, so do not take or increase zinc supplements without the advice of a physician.

132. The first step toward treatment of tinnitus is to go to a doctor to have your ears cleaned. Excessive wax in the ears can make tinnitus worse. Using cotton swabs inside the ear canal can push it up against your eardrum.

133. If you have a wave-like sound in your ears and it's driving you nuts, close your eyes and imagine you're next to the ocean. Each time you hear the whooshing sound, pretend it's a wave lapping up on the beach. If you hear buzzing, picture yourself in a field full of bees.

134. Tinnitus might not be what's keeping you up at night, instead it could be stress which makes the noise more noticeable. Try to tie up as many loose ends as you can before you go to bed and then engage yourself in some relaxation techniques like meditation or deep breathing to clear your mind and calm your body.

135. Use a properly fitted medical device to help relieve tinnitus. A hearing aid alleviates symptoms in about half of tinnitus patients who also have

hearing loss. A "tinnitus masker," a device worn in the ear which produces a low-level noise that helps cover the unpleasant ringing sensation, can also benefit patients without hearing loss.

136. If you suffer from tinnitus, it is important that you avoid stress as much as humanly possible. Stress is very harmful to your body and has a negative effect on all diseases, tinnitus included. Take time to walk and meditate, listen to peaceful music, or participate in any activity that you enjoy and find soothing.

137. When your tinnitus is bad, think about all of the good things in your life. Make a list of everything that you are thankful for, and look at this list whenever you are having a bad day. It will remind you of all the positive things that you have and help to offset the terrible negativity that tinnitus can induce.

138. When you are having a really rough day dealing with your tinnitus, sit yourself down and make a list of everything in your life that is positive. Write about your friends and family and about the people that make you happy. Write about the days when your tinnitus is at a minimum and how you feel on those days.

139. Learn relaxation techniques that promote calm to fight the symptoms of tinnitus. Studies have shown that relaxing activities, like meditation, work to reduce the level of ringing in the ears. Make a deep relaxation routine part of your day to day life. It will not take long to see results.

140. If you have tinnitus, and get it easily, bring some ear plugs along with you. They should be used to prevent exposure to the eardrum from really loud sounds, vibrations, or music that could cause more permanent damage. If you notice a correlation between your tinnitus and a specific place or activity, avoid this trigger if at all possible.

141. Do not let tinnitus get you down. Find something you enjoy doing. If you are really having fun, you will not think about tinnitus anymore and you will not notice it as much when it occurs. You should not dismiss tinnitus as an insignificant issue, the constant discomfort could have a heavy toll.

142. Stress can cause tinnitus. Identify the sources of your stress and do what you can to be more relaxed. Find a hobby to help you relax in your free time and avoid stressful situations if you can. Perhaps you should learn meditation or yoga to help you get rid of your stress.

143.   Do not believe that there is nothing to be done for your tinnitus. If your physician tells you that you will just have to learn to live with it, it is time to find another doctor. New research in the field is offering the medical community a better understanding of tinnitus and new ideas for its treatment.

144.   See if you can track down the most likely trigger for your tinnitus symptoms. Look at everything in your life from your daily habits, to the way you eat, to even prescription medications you just recently included into your body. Things that you eat like sugar, tobacco, alcohol, caffeine, and salt can make tinnitus worse and should be taken out of your diet to see if that is what is causing it.

145.   Be patient when beginning a new treatment for tinnitus. Many treatments require some time before they start working and for results to become apparent. In the meantime, make an effort to eliminate sources of stress in your life as it can often cause the symptoms of tinnitus to become more severe.

146.   Avoiding stress is a great way to keep your tinnitus symptoms at a minimum, but an even better technique is to learn how to cope with stress when it comes up. I like to step back and look at

the situation as if I was a third party, analyzing it and deciding whether or not it's worth my tinnitus acting up. It usually isn't!

147. If you are afflicted with tinnitus, you should consider utilizing techniques that help you relax. Yoga and meditation are two great options. Stress and tension can frequently aggravate tinnitus. Good yoga practice and regular meditation both provide effective tinnitus relief by relaxing the body completely.

148. If you have a wave-like sound in your ears and it's driving you nuts, close your eyes and imagine you're next to the ocean. Each time you hear the whooshing sound, pretend it's a wave lapping up on the beach. If you hear buzzing, picture yourself in a field full of bees.

149. Avoiding caffeine at bedtime is an excellent strategy to employ if you're having trouble falling asleep due to tinnitus symptoms. To begin with, a caffeine allergy can actually cause tinnitus symptoms in healthy individuals, but it will also keep you awake and consciously focused on your tinnitus symptoms at bedtime.

150. Reflexology is a treatment that some tinnitus sufferers have found to be highly effective, so

check it out. Locate an accredited professional with references available. Find someone you can trust and that has experience.

151.   Consider that the source of the ringing in your ears might actually be a problem in your mouth. Have your teeth thoroughly looked at and fix any dental issues. Make sure that any braces, retainers or dentures fit perfectly well and are not tensing muscles further up the head or causing never pains or pinches.

152.   If you are dealing with tinnitus, make an effort to reduce the stress in your life. As with many health conditions, excess stress can make your tinnitus symptoms worse. Take a look at your life to see where the extra pressures may be coming from, and take steps to lighten your load.

153.   If your tinnitus has caused you to have a hearing loss, you should purchase hearing aids. The audible sounds that are produced by these devices can help mask tinnitus when a person is wearing them. For those with profound hearing loss and have little or no hearing, cochlear implants can be very beneficial.

154.   Stay away from loud noises if you have tinnitus. Loud noises will make your situation worse. If this

is impossible for you to do, use ear plugs to drown out some of the noise. It is a good idea to always have ear plugs with you just in case you need them.

155. One method that is effective in alleviating pulsatile tinnitus is removing the ear wax that is impacted in your ear canal. There are several products that can be purchased over-the-counter to remove the ear wax. However, to get the best results in ear wax removal, you should have it removed by a medical professional.

156. Be aware of your unfinished business throughout the early part of the day and try not to leave anything too important on your plate. That way, when you lay down at night, your tinnitus won't be aggravated while you are consumed in thoughts about what you failed to complete throughout the previous day.

157. One sure-fire thing that will make you feel better if you are feeling down in the dumps about your tinnitus is the fact that it could be worse. Tinnitus is something that you can live with. There are many people out there that have been diagnosed with cancer and other life-threatening illnesses. Be happy.

158. Keep busy when you have tinnitus. When you fill up your time with activities, you will not have the time to focus on the ringing in your ears. Go ahead and spoil yourself. Do fun things, and wear yourself out. There is nothing wrong with keeping yourself distracted for the sake of your sanity.

159. Although earwax is important to protect your ears from dirt and bacteria, it is also something that could cause tinnitus. If you get too much of the ear wax built up, it could cause an irritation to your ear drum that could cause the ringing in your ear. So be sure to clear your ears of any ear wax that could have built up.

160. A lot of individuals drink alcohol as part of a celebratory event or as a means of relaxation. Alcohol does, however, encourage dilation in your blood vessels, which causes blood to move with more strength throughout your body. The noise you hear will worsen with the ingestion of alcohol. Coupled with a hangover, you're in for a bad day. Make an effort to reduce or eliminate the amount of alcohol that you drink.

161. Many people have a hard time accepting that they may be suffering from hearing loss. However, if you happen to notice that this may be the case with you or if someone has mentioned something

to you, you should go and have your ears checked. Your tinnitus could be caused by hearing loss and getting a hearing aid can make a difference for you.

162.   Ask your doctor to review the medications you're currently on to see if any of them could be causing your tinnitus symptoms. There are quite a few drugs which can actually bring on tinnitus, so switching that pill for another option can help you to cure your tinnitus and stay healthy with your other condition.

163.   Often it is not the situation itself which is stressful, it's actually how you react to it. Tinnitus symptoms get much worse when you're anxious, so learning tension relief techniques can help you to both feel better about your situation and have your tinnitus reduce in severity during these times.

164.   Bring up your tinnitus to your doctor at your next yearly physical exam and ask to be referred to an ear, nose, and throat specialist. An ENT can look into the cause of your tinnitus, which is vital, if you are going to find a way to treat it.

165.   Join a support group if you suffer from chronic tinnitus. Tinnitus can be extremely stressful for some people, and having someone to talk to about it can help you feel better. It also is beneficial to be

around others that understand what you are going through. If you cannot find a group locally, you can join one online.

166.   While the thought of a 20-minute catnap during the day is appealing, there is no such thing as a nap for tinnitus sufferers. Tinnitus is often linked with insomnia, so a nap will only leave you feeling somewhat groggy and not completely with it, when you try to go to bed for the night.

167.   Stick to a strict sleep schedule. Routine is the best medicine for tinnitus sufferers. Get up in the morning and go to bed at night at the same time each day, including holidays and weekends. This may seem redundant, but it is the key to avoid lying in bed at night awake.

168.   In order to better deal with your tinnitus, try to stay away from loud noise; it will only exacerbate your condition. You may also want to carry earplugs with you in the event that you cannot avoid a noisy situation. If worse comes to worse, you can always use your fingers to block the noise as well.

169.   To stay positive in the face of your condition, seek out a tinnitus support group. It can be difficult for people to understand what you're going

through if they don't have tinnitus themselves. Talking to people who really understand your struggles can be wonderful. If there's not a support group in your area, try to find one online.

170. Reduce your intake of caffeine and salt. Caffeine is a stimulant that not only increases your heart rate but also elevates tinnitus levels. Salt acts similarly by elevating blood pressure and increasing aggravating noise levels in your head. Making dietary changes will reduce tinnitus levels and help you get a better night's sleep.

171. Get a sound generator for your bedroom. The white noise generated by these machines is a great way to defocus your brain, and allow it to take you to dreamland. This allows you to get a peaceful night's sleep.

172. It's said that good dogs are dogs that are tired, and the same can be said for people suffering from tinnitus as well. Being exhausted at bedtime can help you fall asleep much easier. In addition to a host of other benefits, exercise can help alleviate tinnitus symptoms.

173. Having gentle white noise can help you fall asleep when you have tinnitus, but loud noise can sometimes make your situation worse. Keeping

earplugs with you when you travel can help you fall asleep without being kept awake by the parties in the next room or other noisy annoyances.

174. Exercise is a great way to address tinnitus. Not only does it reduce stress, which helps all physical and mental ailments, walking and running in certain environments can really get your mind off the noise. Try going out when it is windy, or by the ocean if you are near one. Any place with constant yet natural sound can give you a pleasant substitute to your tinnitus.

175. Try to do as many interesting and fun things as you can each day. This makes it easier to avoid fixating on the ringing in your ears. Many people let this condition rule their lives, though you do not have to do that. You still need to go out, have fun and, most importantly, keep yourself distracted.

176. Vapor Rub has been proven to help some tinnitus sufferers if your tinnitus is related to sinus, pressure in the head and Eustachian tubes. Some patients have experienced a calming effect on their tinnitus with the use of the vapor rub. It is recommended that you apply some before going to sleep at night for best results.

177.   Although there is limited proof that this in fact works, many people who suffer from tinnitus have stated that various forms of alternative medicine has made a difference for them. Things you might want to consider include: acupuncture, hypnosis, the herb ginkgo, zinc supplements, or lipoflavonoid. Be sure to check with your doctor though before taking a variety of supplements.

178.   The state of your mouth could actually affect the severity of your tinnitus. Make sure you get all dental issues taken care of and ensure you don't have temporomandibular joint disorder as either of those can make your symptoms far worse or even create the problem altogether when you don't have tinnitus at all!

179.   I've had acupuncture a few times in my life and I have to say it was effective for everything I was trying to fix, from speeding up my labor to lessening the severity of my tinnitus symptoms. Find a practitioner in your area who has a sterling reputation and give it a try yourself!

180.   Your dentist might be able to assist if your tinnitus is the result of jaw or mouth problems. One of the possible causes of tinnitus is TMJ, or temporomandibular joint. This is when your jaw is out of alignment. If this is your problem, find a

good dentist who can diagnose the condition and take measures to correct it. This should help to relieve your tinnitus.

181. Consider investing in a quality white noise machine for bedtime. Having some background noise can distract you from your tinnitus and make it easier to sleep. Bear in mind, though, that background noise aggravates tinnitus for some. The only way to tell how it will work for you is to try it for yourself.

182. Research some relaxation techniques, such as deep breathing or meditation. For many people, being stressed can make the tinnitus worse, and the tinnitus itself causes you stress. This positive feedback loop can be broken through the use of relaxation techniques, which can help reduce the incidents of tinnitus in your life.

183. If you believe you might be afflicted with Tinnitus, but you're over 50 you should ask your doctor to test you for Meniere's Disease. This syndrome can afflict you with the same symptoms that Tinnitus can but is far more serious, therefore, a diagnosis is important to help treat it before it gets worse!

184. Spend some money on a good sound generator
and put it very near your bed frame's head. This
sort of generator provides a solid, white noise that
refocuses your thoughts away from the annoyance
of tinnitus sounds. Being able to override the
persistent noise in your ears will allow you get a
good night's sleep.

185. One way to prevent tinnitus from disrupting
your sleep, is to use white noise machines or fans
to drown out the tinnitus sounds. Experiment with
varying background noises to find the type of noise
that is soothing and comforting enough to allow
you to fall asleep. White noise offers a welcome
distraction from the ringing in your ears, which
may make it easier to fall asleep.

186. If you suffer from tinnitus work to relieve any
sinus congestion you may have. The pressure from
congestion can increase your tinnitus symptoms.
Try sleeping with your head elevated and if you
have allergies treat them the best that you can.
Keeping a warm humidifier can also help to open
up the congestion, which will relieve your tinnitus
symptoms.

187. If you are stressed by the constant symptoms of
your tinnitus, it may be time to consider
meditating. Meditation is synonymous with relaxing

the body as well as the mind. A good meditation regimen helps to minimize external and internal distractions. This helps sufferers of tinnitus focus on other things and get a little sleep.

188. If you are dealing with tinnitus, make an effort to reduce the stress in your life. As with many health conditions, excess stress can make your tinnitus symptoms worse. Take a look at your life to see where the extra pressures may be coming from, and take steps to lighten your load.

189. If you have been formally diagnosed with tinnitus, you may be able to decrease its effects by practicing common relaxation techniques. An individual who is placed under a great deal of stress often finds that his or her tinnitus becomes far more intense as a result. Try controlled breathing, stretching, or meditation to avoid making the ringing worse.

190. Make sure you don't have any dental problems. See a dentist and make sure you don't have temporo-mandibular joint disease, or any kind of dental or jaw problem that could be causing your tinnitus. In some cases, taking care of dental issues could alleviate any tinnitus you might be experiencing.

191.   You may find some relief from tinnitus if you just find a good masking noise to listen to. This noise could be a ticking clock, static from an unturned radio or an unturned TV channel. The quieter your surroundings are, the more the noises of tinnitus are going to bother you.

192.   Don't make tinnitus worse by exposing yourself to loud noise. Unexpected noise is always a possibility, so you should always keep earplugs handy to deal with noises you can't get rid of or get away from. No earplugs? At the very least, use your fingers. If you find yourself without earplugs, and in the presence of unhealthy noise levels, simply plug your ears with your fingers.

193.   If you have a continual ringing or buzzing in your ear and think you may have tinnitus, you will need to visit a doctor or other health care provider to set up an appointment for a hearing test. A hearing test can be used to accurately assess your condition. After your hearing test, your health care provider will be able to better evaluate the various factors which might be causing the sounds in your ears.

194.   Tinnitus is often caused by dental problems. Visit your dentist to have him check your mouth. Your bite could actually be what's causing your

tinnitus! If this is the problem, your dentist can recommend treatment to correct the alignment and eliminate your symptoms.

195. If your tinnitus is getting you down you should instead focus on what's great about your life. Write a list of everything you love, enjoy doing, or are happy you are involved in. This will perk up your spirits and help you to get over the misery tinnitus can bring.

196. Some who suffer from tinnitus tout the benefits of ginko biloba, claiming that the plant-based remedy eases their symptoms. Check with your doctor before trying this. No studies have proven how ginko biloba really works, but it is efficient in a lot of cases.

197. There are many factors which can cause tinnitus. Exposure to loud noise, allergies, stress, high blood pressure, and similar factors can make a person experience tinnitus. You should go to a doctor to have them assess your situation and see if they can pinpoint the specific cause. While is is not a disease, it can be diagnosed by your physician.

198. If your tinnitus is driving you crazy, make use of background noise generated by the TV, a fan or any other handy device. Steady noise in the

background can mask the tinnitus, and it may not bother you so much. If the only noise you hear is tinnitus, it's easy to fixate on the sound and become more aggravated by it.

199. Go to sleep in a room that is void of any light. Also make sure to go to sleep with some noise playing in the background. For example, you could leave on some soft music or use a white noise machine. Both of these things will help you get more rest and reduce the symptoms of your tinnitus.

200. There is some evidence out there that shows tinnitus is considered an inflammatory condition. This being said, it makes a great deal of sense to start an anti-inflammatory diet to try to gain some control over your symptoms. A dietary regimen such as this would include plentiful servings of both fruits and vegetables, but also known anti-inflammatories like flax seed oils and salmon.

201. Make a playlist of pleasant music. When you have tinnitus and you want to go to sleep, it can be difficult to fall asleep. Making a playlist of your favorite music and play it as you go to sleep. This will help you to ignore the ringing in your ears.

202. If you are dealing with tinnitus, make an effort to reduce the stress in your life. As with many health conditions, excess stress can make your tinnitus symptoms worse. Take a look at your life to see where the extra pressures may be coming from, and take steps to lighten your load.

203. If you have been formally diagnosed with tinnitus, you may be able to decrease its effects by practicing common relaxation techniques. An individual who is placed under a great deal of stress often finds that his or her tinnitus becomes far more intense as a result. Try controlled breathing, stretching, or meditation to avoid making the ringing worse.

204. Do you have a ringing, hissing, roaring or buzzing sound in your ears that seems to beat in time with your heart? You could possibly be suffering from a condition known as pulsatile tinnitus. Seek advice from your doctor to determine if you are suffering from this condition. Some things that can cause pulsatile tinnitus are excessive ear wax, exposure to loud noises and the stiffening of the bones in the inner ears. By determining the cause for your tinnitus, your physician may be able to help relieve it.

205. One method that is effective in alleviating pulsatile tinnitus is removing the ear wax that is impacted in your ear canal. There are several products that can be purchased over-the-counter to remove the ear wax. However, to get the best results in ear wax removal, you should have it removed by a medical professional.

206. Set a big goal for yourself. Have you always wanted to travel? Do you want to learn an instrument? Place your focus on a future goal and you will be able to distract yourself from the ringing in your ears. Come up with new, more challenging goals and not only will you reach them, you will do so without thinking about your ears.

207. One of the best ways that you can handle tinnitus is to find a support group. This will allow you to meet and speak with people who know exactly where you are coming from and what you are going through. Just knowing that you are not alone can ease the stress of your everyday life.

208. Do not toss out the idea of using a hearing aid. Though it may not be the most fashionable accessory, the ability to hear the things around you is important. You may be surprised at what you have been missing in your daily life. Having one will help you in social situations.

209. Be positive to have the best results in fighting tinnitus. Just focusing on the problem will only depress you. If you are sad about your problems, it actually fuels them and exhausts you since you stay focused about your problems. If you think positive thoughts, you will help your mind stay focused on the positive aspects of life and not controlled by your tinnitus.

210. Visit your dentist. Perhaps you have a problem with your teeth, jaw or skull. Tinnitus that does not respond to treatment should be assessed by a physician. If tinnitus is caused by a physical problem, look into getting things fixed.

211. There's a possibility that you already have a physician, ENT specialist and audiologist, but don't forget that your primary caregiver is you! Only you know exactly how you feel, what your day-to-day life is like, and whether a particular therapy is effective. Your interaction with your doctor and other caregivers is imperative if they are to effectively help in your fight against tinnitus.

212. Try to determine what is triggering your tinnitus. Research the possible side effects of over-the-counter and prescription medications you take on a regular basis to see if tinnitus is listed among them.

Things in your diet including caffeine, salt, sugar, artificial sweeteners, tobacco and salt can make tinnitus worse, so they should be cut, one by one, from your diet to determine if they could be the cause.

213. If you're on pins and needles because of your tinnitus, get a professional to relieve them through more pins and needles! Acupuncture is a great way to heal what ails you, and it can even help with the symptoms of tinnitus. Find a well-respected acupuncturist where you live and give it a try!

214. Learn to control your stress. You can use a variety of methods such as yoga, meditation, support groups, or making sure you get enough sleep. Anything that helps you decrease stress in your life is worth doing. The more stressed you are feeling, the more tinnitus flares up or bothers you.

215. If doctors say they have no way of helping you, keep trying until you find a more knowledgeable doctor. Some physicians are not familiar with tinnitus so they cannot treat it properly, so it is important you go see someone who is well-trained with the condition.

216. Consider investing in a quality white noise machine for bedtime. With the distraction of the

white noise, you may be able to ignore your tinnitus and get some sleep. You may find that this white noise actually exacerbates your tinnitus, though. Try different sounds and see how they work with or against your tinnitus symptoms.

217. Try to avoid exposing yourself to loud noises. Carry earplugs with you for situations where you might be exposed to extremely loud noise. You can even shove your fingers in your ears in an extreme case. For many sufferers of tinnitus, loud noises can trigger or make the condition worse.

218. Seek advice from a doctor if you are suffering from tinnitus. Tinnitus is likely a sign of a different problem that will likely need treatment from a professional. Chronic tinnitus can also be stressful and make it hard to enjoy a normal day. Tinnitus is unlikely to be deadly, but the benefit of seeing a doctor is that it may be treatable.

219. Consider visiting a counselor to engage in cognitive behavioral therapy. The goal of going to therapy is to not focus on you tinnitus. Therapy with a professional helps you to let go of issues, such as anger, that surround your tinnitus. This helps you manage the issue better. You can live a happier life when you are in control of your symptoms.

220. If you are newly experiencing tinnitus, your best approach may be to simply ignore it. The majority of the cases of tinnitus go away on their own. Even if they don't, they subside enough that they do not disrupt your life. If the tinnitus continues to be a problem, however, you should consult your doctor.

221. Many sufferers of tinnitus find it helpful to reduce the stress in their lives. Stress releases chemicals into your body that cause stimulation to your nervous system. Reducing this in your daily life can lessen the symptoms you experience or eliminate it completely. Stress itself could even be the cause of your tinnitus.

222. If you are already suffering from tinnitus, it is mandatory that you take steps now to protect yourself from any further hearing damage. Stay away from loud noises, and wear hearing protection when you cannot avoid noisy environments. Always keep a supply of earplugs with you so that you can take action right away if you find yourself in a situation that could be potentially harmful to your hearing.

223. Help your friends and family to understand what tinnitus is and how it affects you. Let them know what the condition is, what your symptoms feel like

and why certain situations are difficult for you. They will be better equipped to support you if they understand what you are going through and what they can do to help.

224. Whether you have been diagnosed with tinnitus or not, it is nonetheless important that you always use ear protection while in environments that have dangerously high levels of noise pollution. Prolonged exposure to excessively loud noise can increase the likelihood that you will develop tinnitus; it can also cause the condition to become worse in individuals who already battle tinnitus.

225. Find other people who have tinnitus. If you have a network of supportive family and friends, it can reduce your stress and the anxiety that you have about your condition. There are a lot of people who have been through what you're going through, and they can help you by sharing information and helpful tips.

226. When you are having a really rough day dealing with your tinnitus, sit yourself down and make a list of everything in your life that is positive. Write about your friends and family and about the people that make you happy. Write about the days when your tinnitus is at a minimum and how you feel on those days.

227. You should try to go and get your blood pressure checked. Anything from hypertension to other stresses that increase your blood pressure could cause tinnitus to become louder in your ear. If your blood pressure is elevated, try to do things to alleviate it. You should possibly consider taking blood-pressure medication, reducing your caffeine consumption, or just learning different stress management techniques.

228. If you have a continual ringing or buzzing in your ear and think you may have tinnitus, you will need to visit a doctor or other health care provider to set up an appointment for a hearing test. A hearing test can be used to accurately assess your condition. After your hearing test, your health care provider will be able to better evaluate the various factors which might be causing the sounds in your ears.

229. Use background noise to forget about tinnitus. You could leave your TV or radio on, or even hum and sing yourself. Covering the ringing noise will quickly become a habit, and you will soon not even think about tinnitus anymore and simply drown it in other noises. You should be careful about the volume of your background noise.

230. When tinnitus is bothering you, only give yourself about 15 minutes to get to sleep. If you are still awake after fifteen minutes, get out of your bed. Do not engage in any stressful activities. Instead, look for a relaxing activity that will allow you to wind down. By leaving the bedroom, you help make the room a "sleep only" zone. This should, over time, alleviate much of the unwanted tossing and turning you can experience at bed time when you aren't tired enough.

231. Relaxation techniques, like yoga and meditation, can help tinnitus. Stress or tension can worsen the symptoms of tinnitus. To reduce the chances of your tinnitus flaring up, do yoga or meditation to relax your body.

232. In order to better deal with your tinnitus, try to stay away from loud noise; it will only exacerbate your condition. You may also want to carry earplugs with you in the event that you cannot avoid a noisy situation. If worse comes to worse, you can always use your fingers to block the noise as well.

233. Find a tinnitus support group, and attend a meeting. This environment is the right place to get the education you need, as well as the companionship and support from people who

experience the same symptoms as you do. Support groups will assist you in learning how to cope with with the daily challenges of tinnitus.

234.   Try using meditation if you are feeling stressed due to tinnitus and its symptoms. Meditation is known for its superior relaxation techniques. Meditation allows the mind to concentrate and ward off distractions. These types of things can easily benefit any tinnitus sufferer, allowing for an alternate focus and a greater chance for rest.

235.   Many ingredients that are found in popular foods and medications have been shown to irritate the hearing cells. One such ingredient is caffeine, which is a stimulant found in abundance in coffee, sodas, and even in chocolate. By avoiding excessive intake of these caffeinated products, an individual can reduce his or her risk of developing tinnitus or other hearing-related symptoms.

236.   Whether you have been diagnosed with tinnitus or not, it is nonetheless important that you always use ear protection while in environments that have dangerously high levels of noise pollution. Prolonged exposure to excessively loud noise can increase the likelihood that you will develop tinnitus; it can also cause the condition to become worse in individuals who already battle tinnitus.

237. If you begin to suffer from tinnitus, it is important that you remain calm and avoid panic. Remember that tinnitus is almost never a sign of a serious medical condition. Millions of people throughout the world have experienced some form of tinnitus. You are not alone, so stay relaxed and don't be afraid.

238. Use your music or television as a constant background noise to mask out the sounds that you are hearing. If you have other noises going on around you, you will not notice the tinnitus as much, and will be able to function well even when things are getting bad for you.

239. Do you have a ringing, hissing, roaring or buzzing sound in your ears that seems to beat in time with your heart? You could possibly be suffering from a condition known as pulsatile tinnitus. Seek advice from your doctor to determine if you are suffering from this condition. Some things that can cause pulsatile tinnitus are excessive ear wax, exposure to loud noises and the stiffening of the bones in the inner ears. By determining the cause for your tinnitus, your physician may be able to help relieve it.

240. Although there is limited proof that this in fact works, many people who suffer from tinnitus have stated that various forms of alternative medicine has made a difference for them. Things you might want to consider include: acupuncture, hypnosis, the herb ginkgo, zinc supplements, or lipoflavonoid. Be sure to check with your doctor though before taking a variety of supplements.

241. When your tinnitus gets you to your breaking point you should go for a walk! A walk on the beach is an amazing way to cover up the sound while relaxing your mind, but you can also walk through a park or just around the block. Any movement will help you calm down and the tinnitus lessen.

242. I've had acupuncture a few times in my life and I have to say it was effective for everything I was trying to fix, from speeding up my labor to lessening the severity of my tinnitus symptoms. Find a practitioner in your area who has a sterling reputation and give it a try yourself!

243. Do not try homeopathic remedies without talking with your doctor first. Do not try supplements that were not approved by your doctor.

244. If you find that tinnitus becomes a heavy burden to deal with, professional therapy can be very helpful. It not only helps you deal with the negative effects of the tinnitus sounds themselves, but also stress that may be contributing to the problem. You'll find this more than beneficial, if the nonstop ringing in your ears is costing you so much sleep that it's affecting you emotionally.

245. It's extremely important for you to alter the way you treat your ears so that your tinnitus doesn't get any worse! Avoid listening to music at high volume through earbuds, and wear earplugs when engaging in any loud work. You'll want to buy high quality earplugs, not foam, for maximum protection.

246. Make sure you get away from any situations where you're exposed to loud noises. If you can't, such as when you're at work, wear earplugs. Putting yourself too close to noises that are too loud can cause tinnitus or aggravate existing tinnitus problems. Stay away from loud noises in order to stave off any more damage and tinnitus symptoms. It also helps to not bring on an attack of existing tinnitus.

247. Be patient when taking medications to deal with tinnitus. What many tinnitus patients do not realize is that it is common for these medications to take

awhile to settle in, which is why they stop taking them so quickly. It is important to continue taking the medication and you will see positive results, soon.

248. To avoid aggravating your tinnitus further, choose the foods you eat carefully. Salt, caffeine, artificial sweeteners, and sugar, can all make the symptoms of your tinnitus worse. If you don't want to give up all these things, try eliminating them one at a time to find out which one, if any, is causing problems.

249. To get a restful night's sleep even with tinnitus, work out before bedtime. Exercise will tire your body out, and will leave you so exhausted that you'll be able to drift off to sleep peacefully without focusing on your tinnitus. Taking a hot bath after your workout can make falling asleep even easier.

250. There are many natural sleep aids which can help you fall asleep without being harassed by the symptoms of tinnitus. Herbal teas like chamomile are an excellent treatment to start with, but if that doesn't work you can visit a health product store and they'll be able to recommend an item which can provide you with some relief.

251.   Avoid a diet high in sodium to reduce tinnitus symptoms. The more salt you eat, the higher your blood pressure will be, increasing the sound of blood rushing in your ears. Try to eat a healthy diet rich in nutrients and you should experience less tinnitus symptoms.

252.   When tinnitus starts to bother you it's time to get up and do something! Find an activity which can get your mind off the sound, like washing the dishes or running the vacuum. Not only will this help youto get past the annoyance and get back to what you were doing, but you'll leave your home a little cleaner!

253.   Many people who have tinnitus find relief from their condition by utilizing sound therapy. There is a simple experiment that you can try to see if sound therapy will help you cope with your tinnitus. Tune your radio between two stations. You should hear a static sound when you have tuned it between stations. If the static sound from the radio masks your tinnitus or makes it less noticeable (partially masks it), then sound therapy will probably help your condition.

254.   To just live a life free of tinnitus, always have background noise available. Keep a television or music player on. Run a fan. Focus your hearing on

the air conditioning or refrigerator running. Tinnitus is funny in the way that if you do not hear it, it is not really happening.

255.   Many sufferers of tinnitus find it helpful to reduce the stress in their lives. Stress releases chemicals into your body that cause stimulation to your nervous system. Reducing this in your daily life can lessen the symptoms you experience or eliminate it completely. Stress itself could even be the cause of your tinnitus.

256.   Some sufferers of tinnitus have found some relief from their symptoms by using garlic. Garlic has been known to help heart disease, infection and is a powerful anti-oxidant that can even fight cancer. Garlic can be used in the form of supplements found at a health food store, or by using fresh garlic in foods.

257.   You should try to go and get your blood pressure checked. Anything from hypertension to other stresses that increase your blood pressure could cause tinnitus to become louder in your ear. If your blood pressure is elevated, try to do things to alleviate it. You should possibly consider taking blood-pressure medication, reducing your caffeine consumption, or just learning different stress management techniques.

258. Keep earplugs with you all the time if your tinnitus is triggered easily. Also try to avoid areas that are very loud or with intense vibrations. If you find that participating in certain activities, or going to particular places often gives you tinnitus, try to stay away from these locations and activities.

259. In order to treat tinnitus effectively, it is vital that you gather the right team of medical professionals. Ask your primary care physician if she recommends seeing a local ENT or audiologist. If she does, ask her to recommend some good ones.

260. Live your life with an abundance of hope. For someone battling with tinnitus, a chronic condition that leaves your head in a constant state of "noise," your outlook can be very distressing. Hope gives you something to believe in long term, which allows you to feel better both mentally and physically.

261. You may reduce the annoyance factor of your tinnitus by using a source of white noise. Running a fan or other white noise device can help to mask the sounds of the tinnitus and give you some relief. This can be especially helpful at night when you are trying to go to sleep.

262. If you begin to develop any symptoms of tinnitus, you may want to see an Ears, Nose, and Throat Specialist or Audiologist. These two kinds of doctors are trained in dealing with tinnitus, so they would be able to both diagnose the condition as well as properly treat it.

263. To stay positive in the face of your condition, seek out a tinnitus support group. It can be difficult for people to understand what you're going through if they don't have tinnitus themselves. Talking to people who really understand your struggles can be wonderful. If there's not a support group in your area, try to find one online.

264. Reduce your intake of caffeine and salt. Caffeine is a stimulant that not only increases your heart rate but also elevates tinnitus levels. Salt acts similarly by elevating blood pressure and increasing aggravating noise levels in your head. Making dietary changes will reduce tinnitus levels and help you get a better night's sleep.

265. Since tinnitus may be caused by side effects from certain medications, it is important to share with your medical professional all of the current medications you are taking. Be sure to include over-the-counter vitamins, supplements, and

prescription medications to see if any could possibly be the root cause of your tinnitus.

266. If you suffer from tinnitus, your first step should be getting your hearing checked. Even slight hearing loss can be enough to cause an onset of tinnitus. If you find that you do have hearing loss, simply getting hearing aids can eliminate your tinnitus symptoms. In a very few extreme cases, surgery may be necessary.

267. Consider that the source of the ringing in your ears might actually be a problem in your mouth. Have your teeth thoroughly looked at and fix any dental issues. Make sure that any braces, retainers or dentures fit perfectly well and are not tensing muscles further up the head or causing never pains or pinches.

268. It is important to not give up on your tinnitus treatment if it does not seem to be working at first. This is a complex condition that affects a delicate organ of your body. Some treatments can take a while before you start to notice the benefits. Be patient, and give your body some time to heal itself.

269. If you begin to suffer from tinnitus, it is important that you remain calm and avoid panic. Remember that tinnitus is almost never a sign of a

serious medical condition. Millions of people throughout the world have experienced some form of tinnitus. You are not alone, so stay relaxed and don't be afraid.

270. Do you have a ringing, hissing, roaring or buzzing sound in your ears that seems to beat in time with your heart? You could possibly be suffering from a condition known as pulsatile tinnitus. Seek advice from your doctor to determine if you are suffering from this condition. Some things that can cause pulsatile tinnitus are excessive ear wax, exposure to loud noises and the stiffening of the bones in the inner ears. By determining the cause for your tinnitus, your physician may be able to help relieve it.

271. You may find some relief from tinnitus if you just find a good masking noise to listen to. This noise could be a ticking clock, static from an unturned radio or an unturned TV channel. The quieter your surroundings are, the more the noises of tinnitus are going to bother you.

272. Tell your friends and family about what you're going through. It is important for you to surround yourself with people who are understanding and supportive; that can only happen if you share what is happening with your ears. Explain what tinnitus

is, and how it affects your life, so that they are aware and can be there for you.

273.   You should try to go and get your blood pressure checked. Anything from hypertension to other stresses that increase your blood pressure could cause tinnitus to become louder in your ear. If your blood pressure is elevated, try to do things to alleviate it. You should possibly consider taking blood-pressure medication, reducing your caffeine consumption, or just learning different stress management techniques.

274.   Have fun with the sounds you use to cancel out the noise in your ears due to tinnitus! Find all kinds of tracks that help you to feel at peace and negate the ringing, like thunderstorms, music, or the ocean surf. Water is an excellent choice as it tends to mimic the whooshing sound you're hearing.

275.   Avoiding situations which aggravate the symptoms of your tinnitus is an effective strategy to keeping it under control. Stay away from loud noises, stress, caffeine, and sodium-rich foods to avoid triggering your symptoms. Engage in exercise daily to help keep your blood pressure in check and your body healthy to reduce symptoms.

276. Put a high priority on healthy lifestyle choices--
sleep right, eat right, and stay fit. Get eight hours of
sleep everyday, eat healthy food in moderation
several times a day and follow a physical fitness
regimen. Handling the stress of tinnitus will be
simpler if your body is in prime condition. Manage
the basics of life to have a better one, no matter
your level of tinnitus.

277. You might want to visit a specialist who can
determine if you need hearing aids. You may find
that partial hearing loss at certain ranges is
contributing to the unwanted sounds you are
experiencing. Beware though that if the tinnitus
sounds occurs at the same frequency level as that
of the hearing loss that hearing aids may worsen
the condition.

278. Learn to control your stress. You can use a
variety of methods such as yoga, meditation,
support groups, or making sure you get enough
sleep. Anything that helps you decrease stress in
your life is worth doing. The more stressed you are
feeling, the more tinnitus flares up or bothers you.

279. Seek advice from a doctor if you are suffering
from tinnitus. Tinnitus is likely a sign of a different
problem that will likely need treatment from a
professional. Chronic tinnitus can also be stressful

and make it hard to enjoy a normal day. Tinnitus is unlikely to be deadly, but the benefit of seeing a doctor is that it may be treatable.

280.   Research the various natural remedies for tinnitus. There are many means that people were able to successfully treat tinnitus for centuries without the use of medication. Be sure to talk with your physician before trying something, as some herbs can interact with medication, and some of the options available may not be healthy for you.

281.   If you believe you might be afflicted with Tinnitus, but you're over 50 you should ask your doctor to test you for Meniere's Disease. This syndrome can afflict you with the same symptoms that Tinnitus can but is far more serious, therefore, a diagnosis is important to help treat it before it gets worse!

282.   Wash, dry and fold. Not only will doing the laundry keep you busy, but the constant sound from the clothes dryer silences annoying tinnitus ringing. For those who suffer from tinnitus, retraining themselves is a necessary part of helping themselves. By doing a simple household task like laundry, they learn to ignore the agonizing noises in their head.

283. When tinnitus starts to bother you it's time to get up and do something! Find an activity which can get your mind off the sound, like washing the dishes or running the vacuum. Not only will this help youto get past the annoyance and get back to what you were doing, but you'll leave your home a little cleaner!

284. Use your music or television as a constant background noise to mask out the sounds that you are hearing. If you have other noises going on around you, you will not notice the tinnitus as much, and will be able to function well even when things are getting bad for you.

285. If you are having trouble with tinnitus, you may want to try to avoid foods with a good amount of salt or caffeine in them. These foods have been known to agitate tinnitus and if you eliminate these foods altogether, you will have much less of a problem during the day and night.

286. One of the best ways that you can handle tinnitus is to find a support group. This will allow you to meet and speak with people who know exactly where you are coming from and what you are going through. Just knowing that you are not alone can ease the stress of your everyday life.

287. One way to eliminate the stress associated with tinnitus is to repeat your favorite poem. You can do this in your own head or you can scream it from the mountaintops. Have a few favorite poems on hand and repeat them over and over until you feel better and more adequately equipped to do what you need to do.

288. You want to try to limit how often you expose yourself to loud noises. This exposure could be from work-related sounds like chain saws or jackhammers, or it could be from things you enjoy like concerts and MP3 players. So turn down the volume or wear earplugs and protect your ears.

289. Chewing a piece of long-lasting gum can help you to clear out your Eustachian tubes and reduce the severity of the sound in your ear due to tinnitus. I always keep gum handy for times when it's quiet and the noise starts to bother me, so carry a pack with you at all times!

290. I've had acupuncture a few times in my life and I have to say it was effective for everything I was trying to fix, from speeding up my labor to lessening the severity of my tinnitus symptoms. Find a practitioner in your area who has a sterling reputation and give it a try yourself!

291. The many possible causes of tinnitus can make determining the source of your tinnitus difficult. Once you have seen a couple of ear, nose, and throat specialists, it's better to spend most of your resources trying to learn about tinnitus and finding treatments that work for you. Once you have the symptoms under control, you can concentrate on determining the cause.

292. Look into some natural sleep aids that can help you fall asleep at night with your tinnitus. Many of the natural sleep aids are not addictive and can help you sleep in spite of the sounds of your tinnitus. If the natural aids do not work, talk to your doctor about a safe sleep aid you can use.

293. Many people have found relief from their chronic tinnitus from taking nutritional supplements and herbal alternatives. Although there is almost no scientific evidence to back up these claims, people have found some relief using vitamin B complex, mineral supplements with calcium, magnesium, zinc, and herbal extracts like ginkgo biloba.

294. The link between tinnitus and physiological distress requires that a multidimensional approach be used when treating the symptoms of tinnitus. Patient education and coping skills could be

necessary to alleviate the anxiety that tinnitus can cause. Anxiety and stress are common causes of tinnitus and the worry and stress of it can cause it to worsen over time.

295. If you believe you might be afflicted with Tinnitus, but you're over 50 you should ask your doctor to test you for Meniere's Disease. This syndrome can afflict you with the same symptoms that Tinnitus can but is far more serious, therefore, a diagnosis is important to help treat it before it gets worse!

296. The best way to beat tinnitus is to keep positive and upbeat! A happy person tends to be a healthy person, so staying on the bright side of life can help your whole system be in the best shape possible. Stay around positive people, and enjoy life as much as possible!

297. If you are newly experiencing tinnitus, your best approach may be to simply ignore it. The majority of the cases of tinnitus go away on their own. Even if they don't, they subside enough that they do not disrupt your life. If the tinnitus continues to be a problem, however, you should consult your doctor.

298. To just live a life free of tinnitus, always have background noise available. Keep a television or

music player on. Run a fan. Focus your hearing on the air conditioning or refrigerator running. Tinnitus is funny in the way that if you do not hear it, it is not really happening.

299.   Make sure you get plenty of sleep if you are suffering from tinnitus. Chronic fatigue can be a cause of your tinnitus and it can also exasperate the problem. If you have trouble sleeping seek the help of a doctor as your lack of sleep may be the cause of the tinnitus.

300.   Meditation can help relieve tinnitus symptoms that are caused by stress and tension. Meditation reduces both physical and mental stress. More importantly, it helps the brain concentrate on something besides the tinnitus symptoms. This can help those who suffer from tinnitus to finally get some sleep.

301.   Know that you can live with tinnitus. Some people experience tinnitus for just a short time, and others have to learn to handle it daily. You just need to remember that no matter how long you have tinnitus, you can deal with it and live a happy life.

302.   Make a playlist of pleasant music. When you have tinnitus and you want to go to sleep, it can be

difficult to fall asleep. Making a playlist of your favorite music and play it as you go to sleep. This will help you to ignore the ringing in your ears.

303. Multiple studies have shown that elevated levels of blood fats may cause serious and permanent inner-ear malfunction that is accompanied by ringing in the ears. Follow a diet plan that is low in fat; avoid fatty meats, cheeses, fried snacks, and over-processed baked goods. It is not enough to simply avoid trans fats; to protect the health of your ears, you should limit consumption of all kinds of fats.

304. If you begin to suffer from tinnitus, it is important that you remain calm and avoid panic. Remember that tinnitus is almost never a sign of a serious medical condition. Millions of people throughout the world have experienced some form of tinnitus. You are not alone, so stay relaxed and don't be afraid.

305. If the cause of your tinnitus is related to loud noise, it is important for you to wear either ear plugs or ear muffs to protect your ears when you are in situations where there is loud noise. By utilizing these protective devices, you are proactively fighting the chance of serious damage being inflicted on your ears.

306. Figuring out what tinnitus is, and how you come down with the condition, is a great way to go about treating it. You can find many articles, books and websites dealing with the subject. By gaining knowledge about the condition and its causes, you may learn something that can make it more tolerable.

307. Although you do it in silence, Tai-Chi is a great way to relax your body and actually calm the tinnitus that's bothering you. It's an amazing way to center yourself, balance your mind and spirit, and help to keep your blood pressure low. The lower your pressure, the quieter the sound in your ears will be.

308. If you suffer from Tinnitus, make sure to limit the amount of time you spend conversing on your cell phone. It is a scientifically proven fact that long hours spent talking on your cell phone not only results in brain damage, but also worsens Tinnitus. This is important to keep in mind if you enjoy talking on your cell phone a lot. Keep your conversations short and to the point to limit your exposure.

309. Research the various causes and treatments to decrease the symptoms of tinnitus. Read books,

subscribe to blogs and podcasts, and join forums so you can talk with others about how they're treating their disease. You can also put in your "two-cents-worth" regarding your experiences with tinnitus.

310.   You might want to visit a specialist who can determine if you need hearing aids. You may find that partial hearing loss at certain ranges is contributing to the unwanted sounds you are experiencing. Beware though that if the tinnitus sounds occurs at the same frequency level as that of the hearing loss that hearing aids may worsen the condition.

311.   An interesting technique to add to your arsenal in the fight against tinnitus is biofeedback therapy. Often used to help patients reduce their reactions to stress, biofeedback therapy teaches the individual to control certain bodily functions, including their pulse. Many people have discovered that their tinnitus symptoms decrease as they learn to reduce their muscular tension and regulate their skin temperature.

312.   Reflexology is an amazing tool to treat the symptoms of tinnitus. Find yourself an accredited practitioner in your area and ask for references. Then choose the person who you trust and feel

understands your problems the best. In only a few treatments you'll notice that your symptoms will be reduced!

313.

314. There is a small chance that reflexology could help a tinnitus sufferer with his or her symptoms. Always look for professional accreditation and references when you select a reflexology specialist. Do a background check to determine their experience and be sure you can trust them before you hand over any money.

315. To keep tinnitus from driving you crazy, project it out into the room. Visually pick some corner or object in the room you are in and mentally associate that as the source of the sound. If you pretend that it is not within you, then you can mentally relax that there is nothing wrong with you. This improves your mood and blood pressure.

316. To get your mind off tinnitus, create an alternate noise to listen to. Recite poetry or mantras to yourself. Play a musical instrument. You can even chew gum. Singing and humming your favorite songs is always a pleasant way to get through your day and your mind off of the ringing.

317. If you suffer from tinnitus work to relieve any sinus congestion you may have. The pressure from congestion can increase your tinnitus symptoms. Try sleeping with your head elevated and if you have allergies treat them the best that you can. Keeping a warm humidifier can also help to open up the congestion, which will relieve your tinnitus symptoms.

318. Keep calm. Tinnitus is not always related to a major health problem, so calm down so that you do not add stress to your troubles. Worrying will only make you focus more on the tinnitus, which will seem to make it worse. Stay calm and relax so that it is easier to think of other things.

319. Whether you have been diagnosed with tinnitus or not, it is nonetheless important that you always use ear protection while in environments that have dangerously high levels of noise pollution. Prolonged exposure to excessively loud noise can increase the likelihood that you will develop tinnitus; it can also cause the condition to become worse in individuals who already battle tinnitus.

320. When you are diagnosed with a condition such as tinnitus, it is important that you research it and understand it. Make sure to take notes about what triggers tinnitus in you and seek ways of making it

more bearable. Even if the doctor claims that your condition will never go away, rest assured that there are constant improvements in the medical field and there are new cures out there waiting to be discovered.

321. If you are one of the unlucky people that suffer from tinnitus and you have noticed an increase in the severity of it, you may want to have your blood pressure checked. High blood pressure has proven to be one of the causes for increasing severity of tinnitus. If it is high, find ways to lower it.

322. Take up meditation. Meditation will decrease stress, which in turn will make your tinnitus bearable. If you aren't sure how to meditate, start with guided meditations that can help you learn how to relax and enter a meditative state. Learn about the different kinds of meditation to be sure which one is best for you.

323. Something nontraditional that you can do to help with tinnitus is hypnosis. It is not your typical idea, however, is has been proven to help patients in the past. After you are hypnotized by a professional, you can also learn tips and tricks to do self-hypnosis at home.

324. It is a great idea to always carry a set of headphones on you if you have tinnitus. This will protect you from any further damage and will also give you peace of mind if you are in a crowded place with lots of different noises going on around you.

325. Think about buying a hearing aid. Hearing aids may be a solution since they eliminate some of the strain your ears feel. Hearing aids can help you experience normal life by enhancing outside sounds.

326. White noise is used in many places of business for a very good reason. This is because it does a good job of covering up low noises. If tinnitus is keeping you from sleeping at night, you should consider adding some kind of a noise to help cover up the ringing sound you keep hearing. Try turning on a fan, some quiet music, or get a white-noise machine. Is used in many places of business for a very good reason. This is because it does a good job of covering up low noises. If tinnitus is keeping you from sleeping at night, you should consider adding some kind of a noise to help cover up the ringing sound you keep hearing. Try turning on a fan, some quiet music, or get a white-noise machine.